Embracing Healthy Living in The Golden Years

Nigel P Moores

Contents

Preface

When I retired at the age of 65, I was relatively fit, my weight was right and I had never been out of work since leaving school 50 years earlier. I had never had a major illness, indeed I had my first operation at the age of 60 and that was only minor.

So I was looking forward to retirement and having a happy work-free future. However, it wasn't long before I realised old age isn't what it's meant to be, nobody ever warns you, it just suddenly hits you like a rock.

Within a year I was enjoying holidays away, overeating and relaxing on the couch watching TV. I put that much weight on that I got out of breath just going for a walk to the kitchen. My ability to balance was disappearing and my eyesight was a major problem, leaving me visually impaired to the point where I had to stop driving.

I had to do something about it, so I started studying what I needed to do to help me cope with the ageing process. I started investigating ways to get back to enjoying life in my twilight years.

I hope this book allows me to pass on all I learned and in turn enhances the lives of its readers.

So happy ageing everyone and let's show the kids what we are still capable of.

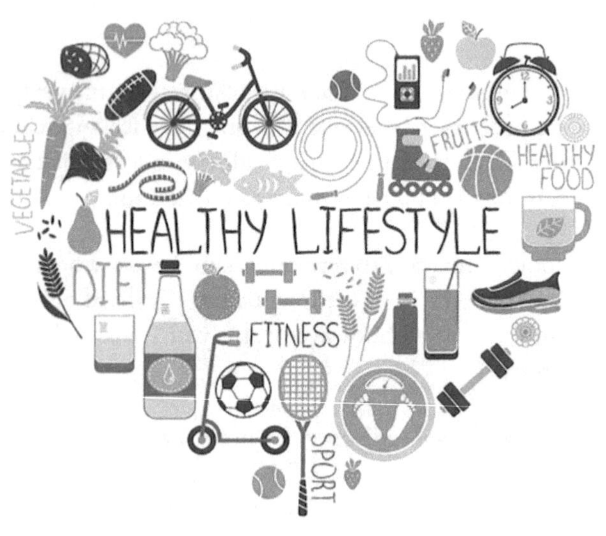

VEGETABLES
FRUITS
HEALTHY
FOOD
HEALTHY LIFESTYLE
DIET
FITNESS
SPORT

Introduction

In the tapestry of life, the golden years signify a period of reflection, wisdom, and the joy of experiences. As the sun sets on one's professional pursuits, it illuminates a path towards a more profound understanding of self and the importance of holistic well-being. This chapter explores the vital facets of healthy living in the golden years, acknowledging the significance of this phase and addressing the common concerns that often accompany aging. Furthermore, it sets the stage for embracing a healthier lifestyle, ensuring that these years are not just lived, but lived with vitality and purpose.

In the twilight years of life, where wisdom finds its home,
A tale of healthy living, in verses I shall roam.
Embracing nature's bounty, in every meal we share,
A vibrant tapestry of colours, a feast beyond compare.

In morning's gentle light, a walk beneath the sky,
Each step a celebration, as years go passing by.
The rhythm of the heartbeat, a song of life's sweet tune,
In every breath, a melody, beneath the golden moon.

With laughter as our medicine, and friendships tried and true,
We find the strength within ourselves, in everything we do.
A dance of joy, a heart that sings, in harmony we're blessed,
In healthy living's guiding light, we find eternal rest.

So let us raise a glass, to these twilight years so dear,
Where health and happiness reside, dispelling every fear.
In every choice we make, let wellness be our guide,
In the twilight years of life, let love and health abide.

CHAPTER 1:

Embracing Healthy Living in the Golden Years: The Importance of Healthy Living in the Golden Years

In the golden years of life, the importance of healthy living cannot be overstated. As we age, our bodies undergo various changes, and adopting a healthy lifestyle becomes crucial for maintaining overall well-being. Healthy living encompasses not only physical fitness but also mental and emotional health. Engaging in regular exercise, consuming a balanced diet, and getting adequate rest are fundamental aspects of healthy living that can significantly enhance the quality of life during the golden years.

Addressing Common Concerns of Aging

Aging often comes with its share of concerns, including reduced mobility, chronic health conditions, and cognitive decline. However, by embracing a healthy lifestyle, many of these concerns can be effectively addressed. Regular physical activity helps improve balance and flexibility, reducing the risk of falls and injuries. Additionally, staying socially active and mentally engaged through hobbies, social interactions, and lifelong learning can enhance cognitive functions and promote emotional well-being.

Moreover, it is essential to address common health issues that arise with age, such as hypertension, diabetes, and osteoporosis. Regular check-ups with healthcare professionals, adherence to prescribed medications, and a healthy diet tailored to specific health needs can aid in managing these conditions effectively.

Setting the Stage for a Healthier Lifestyle

Setting the stage for a healthier lifestyle involves making conscious choices that promote wellness and vitality. It begins with cultivating positive habits, such as incorporating nutritious foods rich in vitamins and minerals into daily meals. A well-balanced diet supports overall health and provides the energy needed for daily activities.

Furthermore, staying physically active doesn't necessarily mean intense workouts; it can include activities like walking, swimming, or yoga tailored to individual abilities. Regular exercise not only strengthens the body but also uplifts the mood and promotes a sense of accomplishment.

Equally important is managing stress through relaxation techniques like meditation and deep breathing exercises. Chronic stress can negatively impact health, so finding healthy ways to cope with stress is vital for emotional well-being. In conclusion, the golden years can be a time of fulfilment, joy, and continued growth when one embraces a healthy lifestyle. By recognising the significance of healthy living, addressing common concerns of aging, and proactively setting the stage for a healthier lifestyle, individuals can navigate this phase of life with vitality and grace.

Embracing the significance of healthy living encompasses a holistic approach to well-being, focussing on physical, mental, and emotional aspects. As we age, common concerns such as declining energy levels, joint pain, and cognitive changes become more prevalent. However, by adopting a proactive mindset and incorporating regular exercise, balanced nutrition, and sufficient sleep, these challenges can be mitigated. Engaging in activities that stimulate the brain, like puzzles or learning new skills, can enhance cognitive function. Additionally, fostering social connections and emotional well-being through meaningful relationships and hobbies can significantly improve overall quality of life.

Furthermore, setting the stage for a healthier lifestyle involves making conscious choices in daily routines. This includes mindful eating, avoiding excessive processed foods and sugar, and staying hydrated. Regular health check-ups, screenings, and immunizations are essential in preventive care. Developing a consistent sleep schedule and managing stress through relaxation techniques like meditation or yoga contribute to overall vitality.

By integrating these practices, individuals can navigate the aging process with vitality and grace. Embracing healthy habits not only extends life expectancy but also enhances the quality of life, allowing individuals to enjoy their golden years to the fullest.

A symphony of processes, both complex and profound,
In the science of living, endless wonders are found.

From the beating of a heart to the sparkle in an eye,
In the secrets of DNA, where our essence does lie,
Life's intricate tapestry, woven strand by strand,
In the study of existence, we begin to understand.

Chemical reactions, like poetry in motion,
Energy transfers, a perpetual devotion,
Cells and organs, harmonising in perfect tune,
In the science of living, there's always something new to learn.

From the microscopic world to the vastness of space,
Life's mysteries unravel, at a steady pace,
In the pursuit of knowledge, we strive to comprehend,
The wonders of life, from beginning to end.

So let us marvel at the science of living, with awe,
For in its exploration, we find the beauty of it all,
A never-ending journey, where discovery takes flight,
In the science of living, we find our guiding light.

CHAPTER 2:

Understanding Aging and Health

Aging is a natural process that every human being undergoes. As we age, our bodies go through various changes, both internally and externally. This chapter explores the science of aging, shedding light on what happens to our bodies as we grow older, the common health issues seniors face, and the importance of addressing mental health and cognitive well-being in the aging population.

The Science of Aging: What Happens to Our Bodies

Aging is a complex biological phenomenon involving gradual, inevitable changes in the body's structure and function. At the cellular level, our cells undergo wear and tear, leading to a decline in their efficiency. This process is influenced by a combination of genetic and environmental factors. As we age, our skin loses elasticity, bones become less dense, and muscles tend to weaken. Internal organs, such as the heart and lungs, may experience reduced efficiency, impacting overall health.

Furthermore, aging affects the brain, leading to changes in memory, cognitive abilities, and processing speed. Neurological conditions like Alzheimer's disease and Parkinson's disease become more prevalent with age, emphasising the importance of brain health in the elderly population.

Common Health Issues Among Seniors

Seniors often face a myriad of health issues, ranging from chronic diseases to age-related conditions. Common health problems include cardiovascular diseases, diabetes, arthritis, osteoporosis, and vision or hearing impairments. These conditions can significantly impact the quality of life for seniors, affecting their mobility, independence, and overall well-being.

Additionally, the immune system weakens with age, making older adults more susceptible to infections and diseases. Vaccinations and proper healthcare management become crucial in preventing and managing these health issues among the elderly.

Mental Health and Aging: Addressing Cognitive Well-being

Mental health is a vital aspect of aging that is sometimes overlooked. Seniors are prone to depression, anxiety, and loneliness, often exacerbated by factors such as social isolation and loss of loved ones. Cognitive decline and dementia are also prevalent concerns, affecting memory, decision-making, and overall cognitive function.

Addressing mental health in the aging population requires a holistic approach. Social engagement, physical activity, and mental stimulation play key roles in maintaining cognitive well-being. Access to healthcare services, counselling, and support groups can provide seniors with the necessary resources to cope with mental health challenges.

In conclusion, understanding the science of aging, being aware of common health issues, and addressing mental health and cognitive well-being are crucial aspects of senior care. By promoting healthy lifestyles, providing adequate healthcare, and fostering social connections, society can help seniors lead fulfilling lives as they age, ensuring their well-being and happiness in their later years.

CHAPTER 3:

Nutrition and Diet

As we age, our nutritional needs change, requiring a more thoughtful approach to our diet. This chapter delves into the crucial aspects of nutrition for seniors, emphasising the significance of a well-balanced diet tailored to meet specific health needs.

Crafting a Balanced Diet for Seniors

A balanced diet for seniors is the cornerstone of good health and vitality. As the body ages, it becomes essential to focus on nutrient-dense foods. Incorporating a variety of fruits, vegetables, whole grains, lean proteins, and healthy fats provides the body with essential vitamins, minerals, and antioxidants. Seniors should pay attention to portion sizes to maintain a healthy weight and prevent overeating.

Importance of Vitamins and Minerals

Vitamins and minerals play pivotal roles in maintaining overall health, especially for seniors. Vitamin D, often called the "sunshine vitamin", is crucial for bone health and immune function. Calcium, another vital nutrient, supports bone strength and muscle function. Seniors should also ensure an adequate intake of vitamin B12, which is essential for nerve function, and vitamin A, necessary for vision and immune system support. Minerals like potassium help maintain healthy blood pressure, while iron is essential for carrying oxygen in the blood.

Special Diets for Seniors (e.g., Diabetic, Heart-Healthy)

Seniors with specific health conditions, such as diabetes or heart disease, must follow tailored diets to manage their conditions effectively. For diabetics, controlling carbohydrate intake, monitoring blood sugar levels, and choosing low-glycaemic foods are crucial. A heart-healthy diet focuses on reducing saturated fats, cholesterol, and sodium while emphasising fruits, vegetables, whole grains, and lean proteins. Consulting a healthcare professional or a registered dietitian can help seniors create personalised meal plans catering to their unique health needs.

Meal Planning and Healthy Recipes

Meal planning is a valuable tool for seniors, helping them make nutritious choices and maintain a balanced diet. Planning meals in advance allows seniors to create well-rounded menus, ensuring they meet their nutritional requirements. Additionally, incorporating healthy recipes into their meal plans adds variety and excitement to their diet. Simple, delicious recipes that feature fresh, whole ingredients can make a significant difference in both the taste and nutritional value of meals.

In conclusion, understanding the importance of a balanced diet, recognising the significance of vitamins and minerals, adhering to special diets when necessary, and embracing meal planning with healthy recipes are fundamental aspects of senior nutrition. By focusing on these elements, seniors can enjoy better health, increased energy, and an improved overall quality of life.

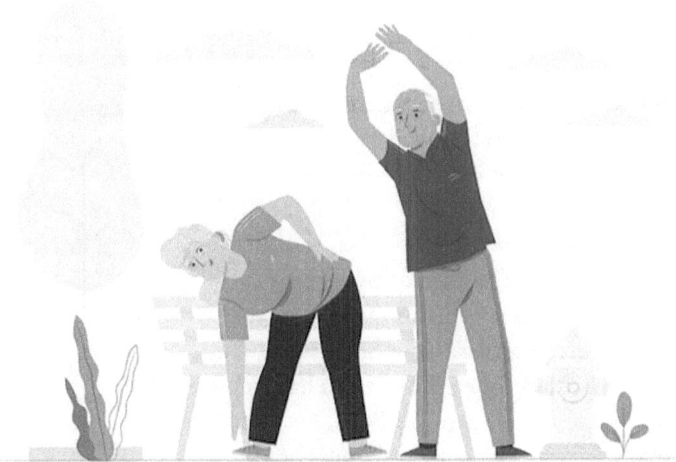

In the realm of motion, where muscles play,

Lies the essence of life in a vibrant display.
Exercise and activity, a harmonious song,
Where strength meets endurance, where we all belong.

With each stretch and flex, the body takes flight,
In the dance of wellness, embracing the light.
Heartbeats drumming to the rhythm of the day,
As we jog, run, or simply sway.

Under the open sky or a gym's bright light,
We challenge ourselves, embracing the fight.
Building our vigour, one step at a time,
In the poetry of movement, so sublime.

In the field, on the court, or by the sea,
We find our solace, wild and free.
Endorphins surge, like a euphoric tide,
In the sanctuary where health and happiness reside.

Exercise, the artist painting colours bold,
On the canvas of life, a story to be told.
Physical activity, a dance of grace,
A symphony of vitality, in every place.

So let us move, let us play,
Embrace the vigour of each new day.
In exercise and activity, we find our might,
A journey to wellness, pure and bright.

CHAPTER 4:

Exercise and Physical Activity

Exercise and physical activity are crucial elements of maintaining a healthy lifestyle, especially for seniors. Tailoring exercise routines to meet the specific needs of older adults can significantly enhance their overall well-being and quality of life.

Tailored Exercise Routines for Seniors

Creating exercise routines tailored to seniors involves considering their individual health conditions, mobility levels, and fitness goals. Low-impact exercises, such as walking, swimming, and cycling, are excellent choices. Additionally, incorporating strength training exercises using light weights or resistance bands can help improve muscle mass and bone density. Balance and flexibility exercises are essential to prevent falls and enhance mobility.

Benefits of Regular Physical Activity

Engaging in regular physical activity offers a multitude of benefits for seniors. Firstly, it improves cardiovascular health, reducing the risk of heart diseases and strokes. Regular exercise also helps in managing weight, reducing the likelihood of obesity and related conditions. Moreover, physical activity enhances mood by releasing endorphins, reducing stress, anxiety, and depression. It promotes better sleep patterns, boosts cognitive function, and strengthens the immune system, leading to an overall improved quality of life.

Yoga, Tai Chi, and Other Gentle Exercises

Yoga and Tai Chi are ancient forms of exercise that are particularly beneficial for seniors. These practices focus on gentle movements, breathing exercises, and meditation, promoting relaxation and flexibility. They improve balance and coordination, reducing the risk of falls. Other gentle exercises, such as water aerobics and stretching routines, are also suitable for seniors, providing a low-impact way to stay active and healthy.

Overcoming Challenges and Staying Active

Seniors may face various challenges when it comes to staying active, such as chronic pain, arthritis, or limited mobility. To overcome these challenges, it's essential to consult healthcare professionals or certified trainers who can design personalised exercise plans. It's crucial to start slowly and progress gradually, listening to the body's signals and avoiding overexertion.

Additionally, social support plays a vital role in maintaining an active lifestyle. Encouragement from friends, family, or participation in group exercise classes can provide motivation and a sense of community. Seniors should also consider using assistive devices like canes or walkers, if necessary, to ensure safety during physical activities.

In conclusion, exercise and physical activity tailored to seniors are fundamental for their health and well-being. By embracing a customized exercise routine, understanding the benefits of regular physical activity, exploring gentle exercises like yoga and Tai Chi, and overcoming challenges with proper guidance and support, seniors can lead active, fulfilling lives, promoting longevity and vitality.

In shadows deep, where silence weaves its song,
A lonely heart, in solitude, is strong.
Amidst the vast and starlit cosmic sea,
A soul finds solace in its reverie.

Through whispered winds, the echoes softly speak,
A dance of stars, a tear upon the cheek.
In solitude, the heart learns to embrace,
The subtle beauty found in empty space.

The moonlight weaves a tapestry of dreams,
Where solitude's not always what it seems.
For in the quiet, there's a strength untold,
A resilience, a spirit to behold.

In solitude, the mind begins to soar,
To places it has never been before.
Embracing loneliness, a cosmic art,
A journey inward, where the soul finds heart.

With every breath, the lonely heart does find,
A peace within, a love of self designed.
Through solitude, a deeper truth is known,
That one is never truly all alone.

CHAPTER 5:

Mental and Emotional Well-being

In the intricate tapestry of human emotions, loneliness and isolation often cast a shadow, challenging the core of our mental and emotional well-being. This chapter delves into essential strategies for coping with these challenges, providing a guiding light toward resilience and contentment.

Coping with Loneliness and Isolation

Loneliness, a universal human experience, can be a formidable adversary. It's crucial to recognise that feeling lonely doesn't necessarily mean being alone. One effective coping strategy involves reaching out to others, whether through social gatherings, community events, or simply a heartfelt conversation with a friend or family member. Moreover, cultivating self-compassion and engaging in self-reflection can foster a sense of belonging within oneself, reducing the impact of external isolation.

Stress Management and Relaxation Techniques

Stress, the silent intruder of peace, requires vigilant management. Stress management techniques, such as mindfulness meditation, deep breathing exercises, and yoga, serve as potent antidotes. These practices anchor the mind to the present moment, fostering tranquillity amidst life's storms. Additionally, embracing a healthy lifestyle through regular exercise, balanced nutrition, and sufficient sleep fortifies the body, enhancing its ability to combat stress.

Pursuing Hobbies and Interests

Hobbies and interests are not mere pastimes; they are lifelines connecting individuals to their passions and purpose. Engaging in activities that spark joy—be it painting, gardening, playing a musical instrument, or exploring the world of literature—not only provides a respite from the demands of daily life but also nurtures creativity and fulfilment. These pursuits stand as testaments to the importance of investing time in activities that bring genuine happiness.

Importance of Social Connections and Support Networks

Human beings are inherently social creatures, wired to seek connections. Building and maintaining meaningful relationships form the bedrock of emotional well-being. Genuine friendships and familial bonds offer unwavering support during challenging times, acting as safety nets that catch us when we fall. Actively participating in social networks, both online and offline, provides avenues for emotional expression, empathy, and understanding, reinforcing the fact that no one has to face life's struggles alone.

In conclusion, mental and emotional well-being are not solitary pursuits but communal endeavours. By acknowledging the challenges of loneliness and isolation, embracing effective stress management techniques, pursuing passions, and nurturing social connections, individuals can navigate the complexities of the human experience with resilience and grace. Remember, in the tapestry of life, every thread of connection and self-care weaves a story of strength and flourishing mental and emotional health.

In the garden of life, where dreams take flight,
Lies a treasure called health, so precious and bright.
With each breath we take, and each step we tread,
Caring for our well-being, our bodies are fed.

A symphony of choices, both big and small,
Nourishing our bodies, minds, and souls, overall.
We sip from the cup of clean water so clear,
Embracing the essence of life, without fear.

In the dance of the sun, and the embrace of the moon,
We find balance and peace, in the morning and noon.
Exercise becomes the rhythm of our beating heart,
A melody of strength, a work of art.

Sleep, a gentle lullaby, wraps us in its embrace,
Restoring our vigour, with each quiet trace.
Vegetables and fruits, vibrant hues on our plate,
Nature's medicine, our health they create.

Mindfulness and joy, like the sweetest song,
Banish stress and worries, making us strong.
Caring for our health, a journey so grand,
Guided by love, with a helping hand.

In the tapestry of life, where stories unfold,
Caring for our health, a tale to be told.
With each mindful choice, and each step we take,
We cherish our well-being, for our own sake.

CHAPTER 6

Medical Care and Preventive Measures

In the realm of healthcare, proactive measures play a pivotal role in ensuring a healthy and fulfilling life. This chapter delves into the importance of regular health check-ups and screenings, the significance of medication management and understanding side effects, the necessity of preventive measures such as vaccinations and fall prevention, and effective strategies for managing chronic conditions.

Regular Health Check-ups and Screenings

Regular health check-ups are the cornerstone of preventive healthcare. By scheduling routine check-ups, individuals can monitor their overall health and detect potential issues before they escalate. Health screenings, including blood pressure, cholesterol, and diabetes/blood sugar checks, enable early diagnosis and intervention, significantly improving the chances of successful treatment.

Medication Management and Understanding Side Effects

Adherence to prescribed medications is crucial for managing various health conditions. Understanding the medications, their purposes, and potential side effects is essential. Patients should maintain open communication with healthcare providers to address concerns and ensure optimal medication management. This knowledge empowers individuals to make informed decisions about their treatment plans.

Preventive Measures: Vaccinations, Fall Prevention, etc.

Preventive measures are vital in reducing the risk of diseases and accidents. Vaccinations protect against a range of illnesses, preventing their spread and safeguarding public health. Fall prevention strategies, especially for older adults, include home modifications, regular exercise, and vision checks, minimising the risk of falls and related injuries. By embracing these measures, individuals can maintain their independence and well-being.

Managing Chronic Conditions Effectively

Chronic conditions require comprehensive management strategies to enhance the quality of life for affected individuals. This involves a multidisciplinary approach, including medical treatments, lifestyle modifications, and emotional support. Patients with chronic illnesses benefit from personalised care plans tailored to their specific needs, ensuring they can lead fulfilling lives despite their health challenges.

In conclusion, prioritising regular health check-ups, understanding medication management, embracing preventive measures, and adopting effective chronic disease management strategies are fundamental aspects of healthcare. By incorporating these practices into their lives, individuals can proactively safeguard their well-being, promoting a healthier and happier future.

In the realm of dreams, where shadows softly creep,
Lies the sanctuary of rest, where souls take a leap.
In the quiet hours of the night, a treasure we keep,
A gift bestowed upon us, the importance of sleep.

Beneath the blanket of stars, the world finds peace,
As weary hearts and minds find sweet release.
In slumber's embrace, all worries cease,
In the tapestry of dreams, our spirits increase.

A healing balm for body, mind, and soul,
Sleep knits the broken, makes us whole.
Through the silent night, it takes control,
Rejuvenating us, making us feel truly whole.

In dreams, we wander, exploring the unknown,
A voyage of wonder, where seeds are sown.
Ideas blossom, creativity is honed,
In the realm of sleep, inspiration is shown.

So close your eyes, let go of the day,
Embrace the night, let sleep guide your way.
For in its embrace, we find our say,
The importance of sleep, in every way.

CHAPTER 7:

Sleep and Rest

Quality sleep is crucial for individuals of all ages, but it holds particular significance for seniors. In this chapter, we will delve into the importance of quality sleep for seniors, explore common sleep disorders affecting this demographic, and discuss effective strategies for creating a relaxing bedtime routine.

Importance of Quality Sleep for Seniors

As we age, our bodies undergo various changes, including alterations in sleep patterns. Quality sleep plays a vital role in maintaining good health and well-being for seniors. Adequate sleep enhances cognitive function, boosts the immune system, and promotes emotional stability. For seniors, quality sleep is essential for memory consolidation, learning, and overall brain health. Moreover, it aids in muscle repair, reduces inflammation, and contributes to a lower risk of chronic diseases such as diabetes and heart conditions.

Addressing Sleep Disorders

Seniors are often prone to sleep disorders, including insomnia, sleep apnoea, restless leg syndrome, and periodic limb movement disorder. These disorders can significantly impact the quality of sleep, leading to daytime fatigue and decreased overall well-being.

Insomnia

Insomnia, characterised by difficulty falling or staying asleep, can be caused by various factors such as medication, chronic pain, or stress. Seniors should consult healthcare professionals to identify the underlying cause and explore suitable treatments, which may include therapy, lifestyle changes, or medications.

Sleep Apnoea

Sleep apnoea, a condition where breathing stops and starts during sleep, is common among seniors. Continuous positive airway pressure (CPAP) machines are often prescribed to help maintain steady breathing patterns, ensuring uninterrupted sleep.

Restless Leg Syndrome and Periodic Limb Movement Disorder

Restless leg syndrome and periodic limb movement disorder involve repetitive movements of the legs during sleep, leading to disrupted sleep. Treatment options may include medications or lifestyle adjustments to alleviate symptoms and improve sleep quality.

Creating a Relaxing Bedtime Routine

Establishing a calming bedtime routine can significantly enhance sleep quality for seniors. Here are some effective strategies:

1. Limit Stimulants: Avoid caffeine and nicotine in the hours leading up to bedtime, as these substances can interfere with sleep.

2. Create a Comfortable Sleep Environment: Invest in a comfortable mattress and pillows. Ensure the bedroom is cool, dark, and quiet. Consider using blackout curtains and white noise machines to create an ideal sleep environment.

3. Establish a Regular Sleep Schedule: Aim to go to bed and wake up at the same time every day, even on weekends. Consistency reinforces the body's natural sleep-wake cycle.

4. Relaxation Techniques: Engage in relaxation activities such as reading, gentle stretching, or deep breathing exercises before bedtime. These activities can help calm the mind and prepare the body for sleep.

5. Limit Screen Time: Reduce exposure to electronic devices like smartphones and computers before bedtime. The blue light emitted by these devices can interfere with the production of melatonin, a hormone that regulates sleep.

In conclusion, prioritising quality sleep and addressing sleep disorders are essential aspects of senior healthcare. By incorporating these strategies and creating a relaxing bedtime routine, seniors can enjoy restful nights, leading to improved overall health and well-being.

CHAPTER 8:

Financial and Legal Planning

In today's fast-paced world, financial and legal planning are essential aspects of a secure and comfortable future. This chapter explores the intricacies of financial planning, retirement strategies, and the importance of legal documents, shedding light on how individuals can safeguard their assets and well-being.

Retirement Planning and Budgeting

Retirement planning is a cornerstone of financial stability. It involves thoughtful consideration of one's financial goals, lifestyle expectations, and the steps required to achieve them. Budgeting, a crucial component of this process, allows individuals to track their income and expenses, ensuring a balanced financial life. By saving consistently and investing wisely, individuals can create a nest egg that supports them during their retirement years, providing financial freedom and peace of mind.

Healthcare and Insurance Options

Healthcare and insurance are vital aspects of any financial plan. Understanding the available healthcare options, including insurance coverage and savings accounts, is essential for managing unexpected medical expenses. Health insurance provides a safety net, covering the costs of medical treatments and prescriptions. Additionally, individuals can explore various insurance policies, such as life insurance and disability insurance, to protect their families and assets in case of unforeseen events.

Legal Documents: Wills, Power of Attorney, Living Will

Creating legal documents is a proactive step towards ensuring one's wishes are respected, especially during challenging times. A **Will** outlines how a person's assets will be distributed after their passing, offering clarity to family members and reducing potential conflicts. **Power of Attorney** grants a trusted individual the authority to make financial and legal decisions on behalf of the person, ensuring their affairs are managed effectively if they become incapacitated. A **Living Will**, on the other hand, outlines an individual's healthcare preferences, guiding medical professionals and family members in making critical decisions if the person is unable to communicate their wishes.

Understanding the nuances of these legal documents is essential. Consulting legal professionals and financial advisors can provide personalised guidance, ensuring these documents align with an individual's unique circumstances and desires.

In conclusion

Financial and legal planning empowers individuals to take control of their future. By diligently saving, investing wisely, and securing the appropriate legal documents, individuals can navigate life's uncertainties with confidence, knowing they have laid a strong foundation for themselves and their loved ones.

In a world of wires and glowing screens,
Where virtual reality meets our dreams,
We venture forth with hearts alight,
Engaging in the digital flight.

With fingertips that dance and glide,
We navigate the electronic tide,
Through cyberspace, we swiftly roam,
In the realm of ones and zeros, we find our home.

Gadgets and gizmos, they surround,
Innovations that astound,
We connect, we share, we learn, we play,
In the tech-filled dawn of a new day.

Yet amidst the circuits and coded speech,
Let not our humanity be breached,
For in this digital tapestry,
Lies the essence of our shared humanity.

With every click and every tap,
We bridge the gaps, we fill the gap,
Through screens, we find our souls entwined,
In the vast expanse of the digital mind.

So let us embrace this tech-filled age,
With wonder, joy, and mindful sage,
For in engaging technology's embrace,
We discover a boundless, virtual space.

CHAPTER 9:

Embracing Technology

In today's rapidly evolving world, embracing technology has become essential, especially for seniors seeking to enhance their lives and stay connected with the changing times. This chapter explores various aspects of integrating technology into the lives of seniors, ranging from health monitoring to building intergenerational relationships.

Technology for Health Monitoring

The advent of smart devices and health apps has revolutionised healthcare, allowing seniors to monitor their well-being conveniently. From wearable fitness trackers to smartphone apps that track vital signs, technology enables proactive health management. Regular monitoring empowers seniors to make informed decisions about their lifestyle and seek timely medical attention when needed.

Social Media and Staying Connected

Social media platforms offer seniors a gateway to stay connected with friends and family, irrespective of geographical distances. Through platforms like Facebook and Instagram, they can share experiences, photos, and messages, fostering meaningful connections and reducing feelings of isolation. Online communication tools like video calls further bridge the gap, providing a sense of presence despite physical distances.

Learning New Skills Online

The internet is a vast treasure trove of knowledge and learning opportunities. Seniors can explore online courses and tutorials tailored to their interests, allowing them to acquire new skills, hobbies, or even pursue academic interests. Platforms like YouTube offer a plethora of resources, enabling continuous learning and personal growth.

Community Engagement and Volunteering

The digital landscape has transformed community engagement and volunteering efforts. Seniors can participate in virtual community events, town hall meetings, and support groups from the comfort of their homes. Online platforms facilitate volunteering opportunities, allowing them to contribute their skills and experiences to various causes, thereby fostering a sense of purpose and fulfilment.

Participating in Community Events and Activities

Local community events and activities have also embraced technology, offering seniors the chance to participate in virtual workshops, book clubs, art exhibitions, and fitness classes. These events not only provide entertainment but also create a sense of belonging, reinforcing the importance of social connections in the digital age.

Volunteering Opportunities for Seniors

Volunteering not only benefits the community but also enriches the lives of seniors. Many organisations offer virtual volunteering opportunities, such as online tutoring, mentoring, or assisting non-profits with administrative tasks. Seniors can leverage their skills and expertise to make a difference, finding purpose and fulfilment in giving back to society.

Building Intergenerational Relationships

One of the significant advantages of technology is its ability to bridge generational gaps. Seniors can engage with younger generations through online platforms, sharing experiences, wisdom, and stories. Intergenerational relationships foster mutual understanding, respect, and empathy, enriching the lives of both seniors and younger individuals.

In conclusion, embracing technology empowers seniors to lead fulfilling lives, stay connected, and actively contribute to their communities. By harnessing the power of digital technology.

In the golden embrace of aging's grace,
Where wrinkles weave tales on a time-worn face,
There lies a beauty, deep and true,
In every moment life renews.

With silver strands, like moonlight's kiss,
Wisdom blooms in hearts amiss,
Embracing years, we find our way,
Through laughter, tears, come what may.

The lines that etch upon our skin,
Tell stories of the battles within,
A tapestry of moments lived,
In every smile, in every quirk, we're gifted.

With each passing day, we learn to see,
The beauty in life's sweet decree,
In laughter shared, and friendships true,
Embracing the joys of aging, we renew.

For time, it weaves a tapestry,
Of memories, love, and legacy,
In every wrinkle, there's a tale,
Of resilience, and how we prevail.

So let us celebrate the years,
Embracing life, conquering fears,
For in the journey of growing old,
We find a love that's pure, untold.

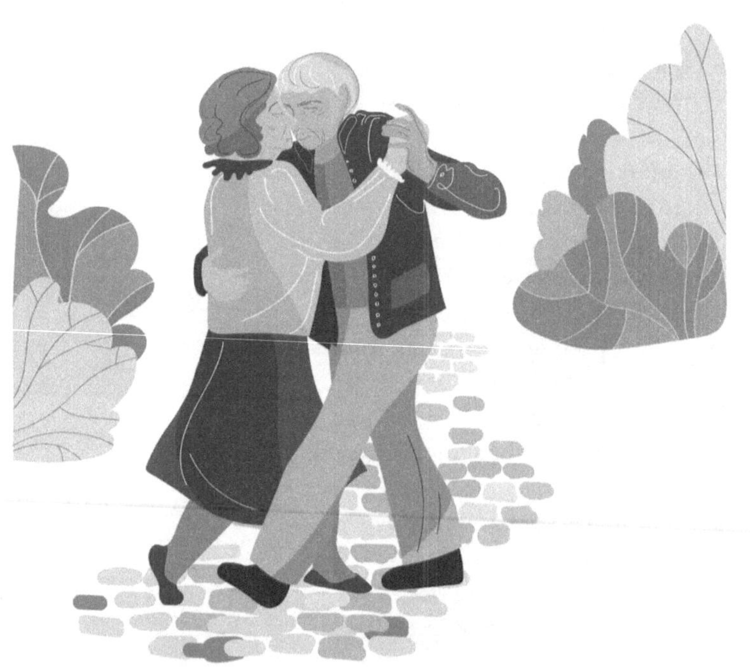

CHAPTER 10:

Embracing the Joys of Aging and Living a Healthy Life

Conclusion

In the final chapters of our journey through life, it becomes imperative to celebrate the joys of aging, embrace a healthy lifestyle, and reflect upon the wisdom and inspiration gained along the way. The essence of a fulfilling life lies not just in the number of years we live, but in how we live those years. This conclusion explores the beauty of growing older, the importance of maintaining one's health, and the profound wisdom that comes with a life well-lived.

Celebrating the Joys of Aging

Aging is not a curse, but a privilege denied to many. As the years pass, we accumulate experiences, memories, and a profound understanding of the world. Every wrinkle tells a story, and every grey hair symbolizes the wisdom gained. It's a time to cherish the moments spent with loved ones, appreciate the beauty of nature, and find contentment in simplicity. Celebrating the joys of aging means embracing the freedom that comes with accepting oneself wholly and finding fulfilment in the little things that life offers.

Encouragement to Embrace a Healthy Lifestyle

Maintaining good health is the key to enjoying the golden years to the fullest. Embracing a healthy lifestyle involves a balanced diet, regular exercise, mental stimulation, and meaningful social connections. It's about nourishing the body, mind, and soul. Engaging in physical activities like walking, yoga, or swimming can keep the body agile and the mind sharp. Cultivating hobbies, learning new skills, and staying socially active can provide a sense of purpose and fulfilment. Making healthy choices not only adds years to life but also life to years.

Final Words of Wisdom and Inspiration

In the tapestry of life, every thread represents a lesson learned, a challenge overcome, or a moment of joy. As we approach the twilight years, it's essential to share the wisdom garnered with the generations to come. These final words serve as a beacon of inspiration, guiding others on their life journeys. Remember that life is a continuous learning process, and every setback is an opportunity for growth. Find joy in giving back to the community, nurture relationships, and never stop exploring the wonders of the world.

In conclusion, embracing the joys of aging, adopting a healthy lifestyle, and sharing words of wisdom are the cornerstones of a fulfilling life. As we celebrate the richness of our experiences, let us inspire others to lead lives filled with purpose, gratitude, and boundless enthusiasm. May the sunset years be as vibrant and meaningful as the dawn, as we continue to learn, grow, and cherish every precious moment life offer. Embracing the joys of aging allows us to appreciate the beauty of life's natural progression, finding fulfilment in the wisdom that comes with each passing year. Adopting a healthy lifestyle becomes paramount, nurturing our bodies and minds to ensure longevity and vitality. Sharing words of wisdom becomes a gift, passing down the lessons learned, shaping future generations with the pearls of our experiences.

Together, these cornerstones pave the way for a fulfilling life, one where purpose, gratitude, and boundless enthusiasm guide our actions. Through this journey, we inspire others, creating a ripple effect of positivity and fulfilment. As the sun sets, let us embrace the twilight years with vibrancy and meaning, savouring every moment and continuing to learn, grow, and cherish the precious gi

When it comes to promoting healthy living, worksheets and checklists can be helpful tools. Here are some ideas for creating worksheets and checklists related to healthy living:

1. Meal Planning Worksheet
   - Plan your meals for the week, including breakfast, lunch, dinner, and snacks.
   - Create a grocery list based on your meal plan, focusing on nutritious foods.

2. Exercise Routine Checklist:
   - Design a weekly exercise routine including cardio, strength training, and flexibility exercises.
   - Create a checklist to track your daily or weekly workouts.

3. Sleep Log Worksheet:
   - Monitor your sleep patterns by recording your bedtime, wake-up time, and quality of sleep.
   - Note any factors that might affect your sleep, such as caffeine intake or screen time before bed.

4. Stress Management Checklist:
   - List various stress-relieving activities like meditation, deep breathing, yoga, or hobbies.
   - Check off the activities you engage in each day to manage stress effectively.

5. Hydration Tracker:
   - Keep track of your daily water intake to ensure you stay properly hydrated.
   - Set a goal for the number of glasses or litres you aim to drink each day.

6. Mental Health Worksheet:
   - Reflect on your emotions, thoughts, and triggers throughout the day.

- Practice mindfulness and jot down positive aspects of your day to promote mental well-being.

7. Healthy Habits Checklist:
   - Include habits like brushing teeth, flossing, and washing hands to maintain overall health.
   - Use a checklist format to ensure you're consistently following these habits.

8. Goal Setting Worksheet:
   - Set specific, measurable, achievable, relevant, and time-bound (SMART) goals related to your health.
   - Break down larger goals into smaller, actionable steps to track your progress.

Remember, these worksheets and checklists can be customised to suit your specific needs and preferences. Feel free to design them in a way that aligns with your goals for a healthier lifestyle!

9 7 9 8 8 7 3 8 5 2 4 5 1